Well-being After Birth

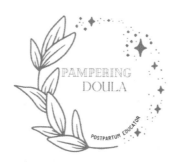

ZAURE VUK

&

ASHLEE SAKAISHI WILKIN

Table of Contents

"Planning for the weeks after birth is so often NOT on the radar of families I work with. It was certainly not where my attention was when I became a mother for the first time. A guide such as this is invaluable for helping expecting parents think about vital support aspects BEFORE they are needed. I love Zaure's guide for the thoughtful organization she invites parents to complete as a way to ensure they are cared for in many ways during the vulnerable first weeks with their babies. We all just need a little guidance! This guide is just that."

Christine Devlin Eck, Ayurvedic postpartum doula educator, founder of the Center for Sacred Window Studies

"This is the guide I wish I would have had when I was preparing for the births of my girls. With much wisdom and grace, Zaure leads expectant mothers through a step-by-step process to prepare for a very vulnerable season. This guide is sure to relieve you from confusion and being overwhelmed by bringing clarity and intention around planning for postpartum."

Amie Cazel, a NYC-based actress, educator, mama of two

"This Postpartum Guide is immensely helpful for anyone who is pregnant. The guide is comprehensive and covers all the vital things new parents need to be thinking about for optimal healing and enjoyment of their postpartum period."

The Doula Darcy, Founder of Doula Business Academy, Doula Business Coach Dover, NH

"Zaure has created a truly beautiful postpartum guidebook for all families going through the journey themselves and all who are serving these families.
Not only is it full of wisdom but you can feel her love and compassion pouring through her words. I highly recommend her guide and creating a supportive container for yourself as you go through the sacred window of postpartum."

Corinne Andrews, mama of two, author of "Birthing Mama: Your Companion for a Holistic Pregnancy Journey", developer/lead teacher of the 90-hour Birthing Mama Prenatal & Postnatal Yoga and Wellness Teacher Training and 200-hour Shraddh⍰

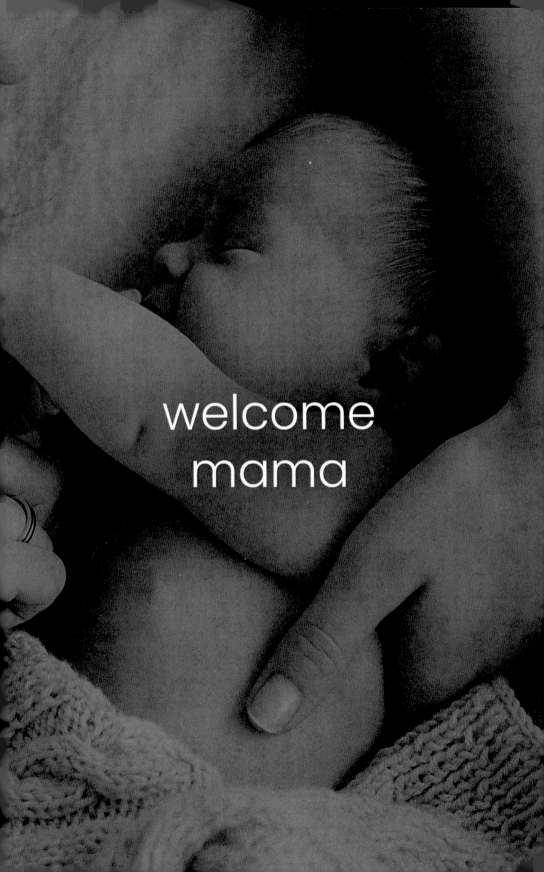

welcome
mama

Welcome to this space, dear Mama,

Does planning for your postpartum window feel daunting?

Do you feel overwhelmed thinking of how many baby bottles to buy, what stroller to choose, or how many boxes of diapers you should have in stock?

Or do you not feel like postpartum time, the first few weeks after birth, needs special planning?

Maybe you think it will be an idyllic, blissful, Pinterest-like time with a newborn who will sleep when you need a break and wake up smiling when you are ready to engage with them again.

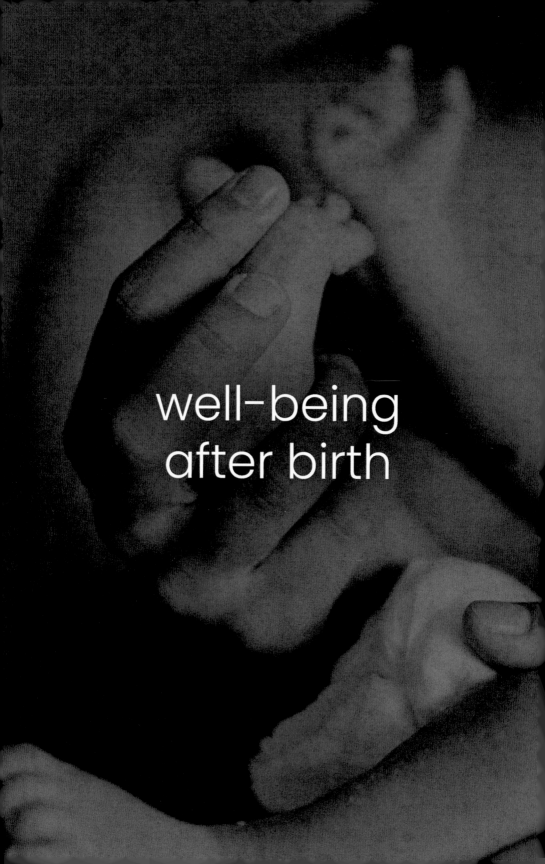

well-being
after birth

Well-being After Birth

This guide is a collaborative work of two professionally trained postpartum doulas and moms who dedicated their work to supporting and nurturing newborn mothers during the first few weeks or months after birth of the baby.

This guide will introduce you to some of the very important needs new mothers experience after having a baby.

If you are planning to have a baby or just had a baby, this guide will give you a great start in planning the care you will need for you and your newborn.

Throughout the Guide, you will read the voices of experts in the field of women's health. They either speak to the physiological needs of the new mother, emotional aspects, or psychological shifts that happen to women due to childbirth.

On these pages, you will see the word **"postpartum."** Very often it is also called **the fourth trimester**, implying the pregnancy period is not actually over with the birth of the baby.

Postpartum is the period of the **first 6-8 weeks after birth**. It is considered to be a very sensitive window of time when a lot is going on in the mother and in the baby.

The environment and the system of support that is created will either help lay a strong foundation for all of the aspects of motherhood and create a strong bonding between you and the baby, or the lack of it can contribute to possibly a traumatic experience that will have an effect for years to come.

> " First of all, you are going to need a lot more help than you think you will need. We tend to think that if we can do something ourselves, then we should. This is absolutely not true postpartum. All of your energy needs to go toward healing your body and learning about your baby. Just as you are providing unlimited food for baby, you need someone to be nourishing you. "

The Fourth Trimester,
Kimberly Ann Johnson

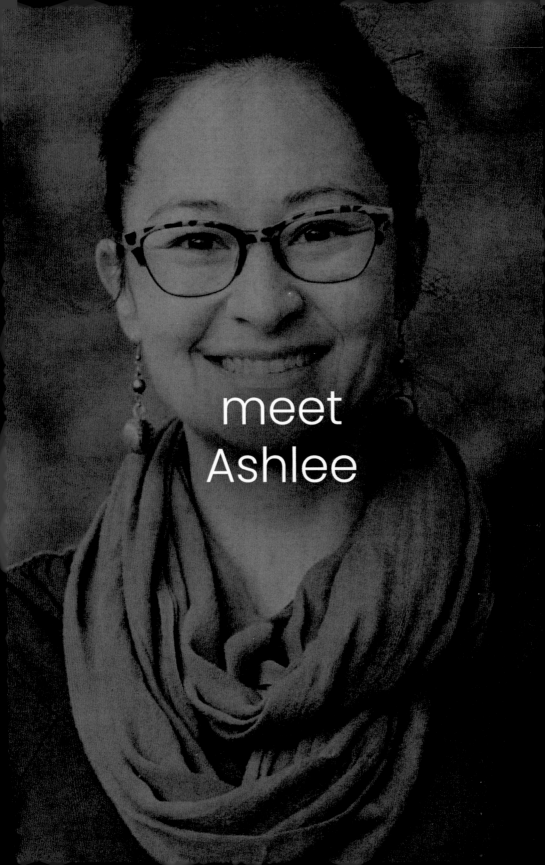

meet
Ashlee

Meet Ashlee Sakaishi Wilkin

> *You will go through a range of emotions that you have never experienced, sometimes all in one day. You will experience periods of doubt. You will need companionship that you can rely on, assuring you that everything is okay, that you will reemerge... I have never heard a woman lament having too much postpartum support. I have only heard women regret that no one told them they should have invested more resources in postpartum care.*

Fourth Trimester, *Kimberly Ann Johnson*

Hi, I am Ashlee. I became a mother in 2019 after a beautiful pregnancy and a challenging three-day induction leading to my son's birth via cesarean. I loved being pregnant and was excited to experience birth, postpartum, and motherhood for the first time.

I had been figuring out what works, what was needed, and how a family could best be supported in parenthood over the previous seven years. I was looking forward to creating a village of support around me so I could experience my own Sacred Window or time of transformation.

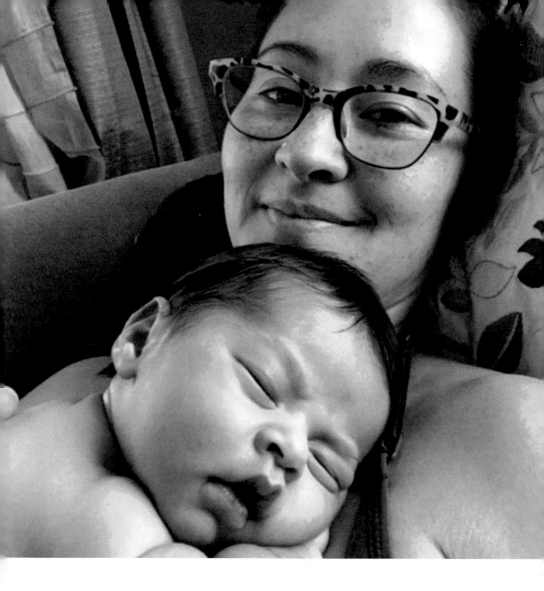

One of the challenges I continue to see is a lack of planning for postpartum and, most importantly, a lack of support for new families in the first two years of their babies' lives.

This guide is a collaborative beginning and a valuable resource for new families to develop and grow connection, community, nourishment, and support as part of their postpartum plan for lifelong health and community.

I was drawn to this work through a love of food, Ayurveda, the powerful transition of maiden to mother, and the opportunity to shift our culture toward a more loving, connected, and supportive family-centered culture. I have worked with families throughout the United States since 2012 as an Ayurvedic Practitioner, Massage Therapist, educator, community activist, and labor and postpartum doula.

I have recognized the challenges and struggles present across geographic locations, family structures, and cultural paradigms for mothers, birthers, and families in the immediate weeks, months, and early years after a baby is born.

I deeply recognize the value of continuing to connect with other new parents in the same stage of postpartum for camaraderie and ongoing support and connection as well as ensuring new parents have a solid postpartum plan in place so they can rest, heal, connect, and be present with their growing family. May you be nourished, may you be healthy, and may you feel connected to the community.

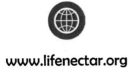

www.lifenectar.org

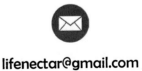

lifenectar@gmail.com

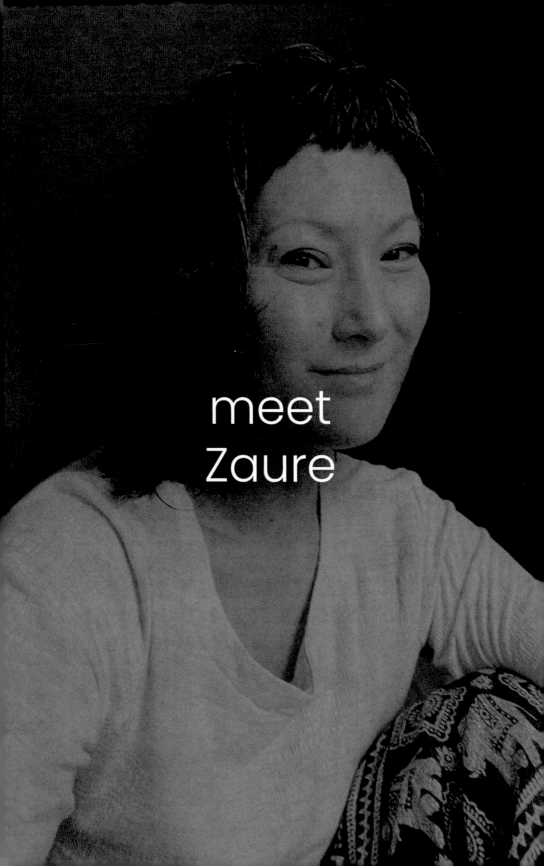

meet
Zaure

Meet Zaure

Hi, I am Zaure. I am a mother of 4, a postpartum doula, and thought that pregnancy and becoming a mother is just a natural process and does not need any preparation or planning. I thought postpartum would be an easy breezy time for me, and I did not need any preparation.

How far from the truth that was. The lack of preparation and planning for postpartum well-being and care for me still has consequences on my health a decade later.

> *What would it be like to feel like a queen, to have your favorite healthy meals cooked and served to you, to have someone else doing the laundry and straightening up the house, to have a massage every week, physical therapy, and dreamy periods of sleep throughout the day with your best girlfriends and relatives around whenever you need them?*
>
> **Although receiving this kind of help seems like a luxury for most of us, postpartum is a necessity.**
>
> Fourth Trimester, *Kimberly Ann Johnson*

I am a mother of four young children. I had three pregnancies, one of which was with twins. Each time I had a baby, or babies, I felt that this huge life transition was not honored or supported as it should be.

When I first had my daughter, I was quite shocked at how isolated and foreign I felt. I am an immigrant, and where I come from new mothers rest for 40 days with their newborns. They are cared for and pampered, and no negativity or sad news is allowed to enter the sanctuary of the mother and her baby. Maternity leave lasts three years, and most mothers stay home caring for the child for at least a year.

I had expected the same level of care and gentleness around me. However, being in America, my experience turned out to be a very traumatic one.

At first, I thought the difference in cultures between America and Kazakhstan did not mean that it was bad. I tried to assimilate into a new country and accept the reality of a lonely and unsupported postpartum.

But then, I had my mom come to help me after my twins were born. And I saw that it can, and in fact, must be different. My mother bathed me, massaged me, took care of the twins, and cooked three times a day, mostly soups, to make sure I was getting nurtured inside and out. This drastic difference in my experiences postpartum changed everything for me. This helped me experience more peace, feel more grounded, and enjoy the time with my babies. I was more resourced and my nervous system was much less taxed with two babies than I felt when I had just one baby before.

As you read the pages of the **Well-being After Birth Guide's pages**, please bear in mind that investing time, energy, and possibly even

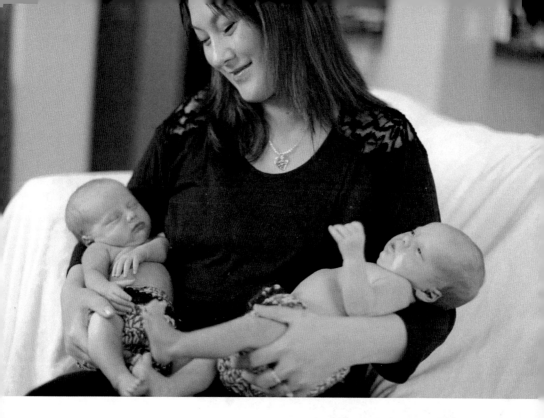

finances in planning your postpartum transition will help your well-being. In turn, you feeling well will directly affect your baby's well-being.

If you are cared for and your needs are met, there are much better chances that you will be better equipped to care for your baby, who is completely dependent on you. The right support from your community, family, and a trained professional postpartum doula will help create a gentle and sacred approach during this sensitive time in your life. These resources, if planned and organized, will set you up to experience transition into motherhood as a meaningful and rich experience.

www.pamperingdoula.com

zaurevuk@gmail.com

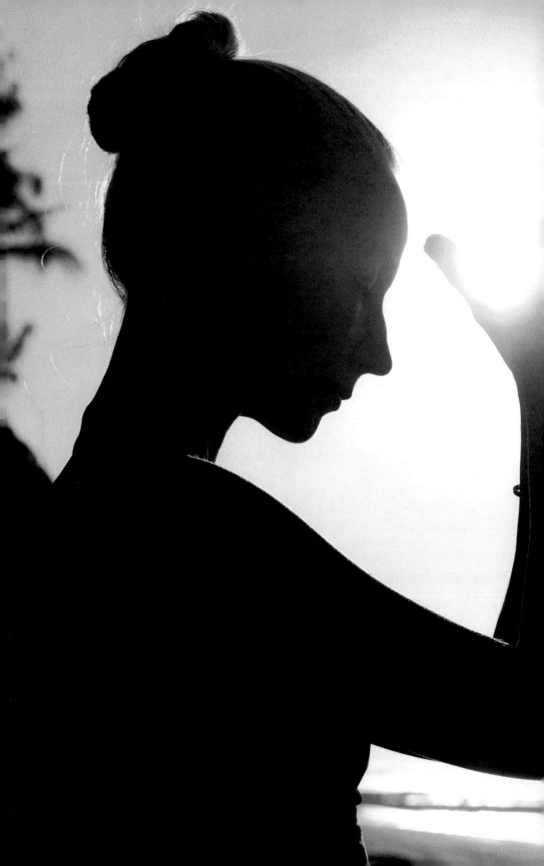

> What is woman's place at this stage of our cultural development? I feel strongly that it is to heal the split that tells us that our knowings, wishes, and desires are not as important nor as valid as those of the dominant male culture. Our task is to heal the internal split that tells us to override the feelings, intuition, and dream images that inform us of the truth of life. We must have the courage to live with paradox, the strength to hold the tension of not knowing the answers, and the willingness to listen to our inner wisdom and the wisdom of the planet, which begs for change.

The Heroine's Journey,
Maureen Murdock

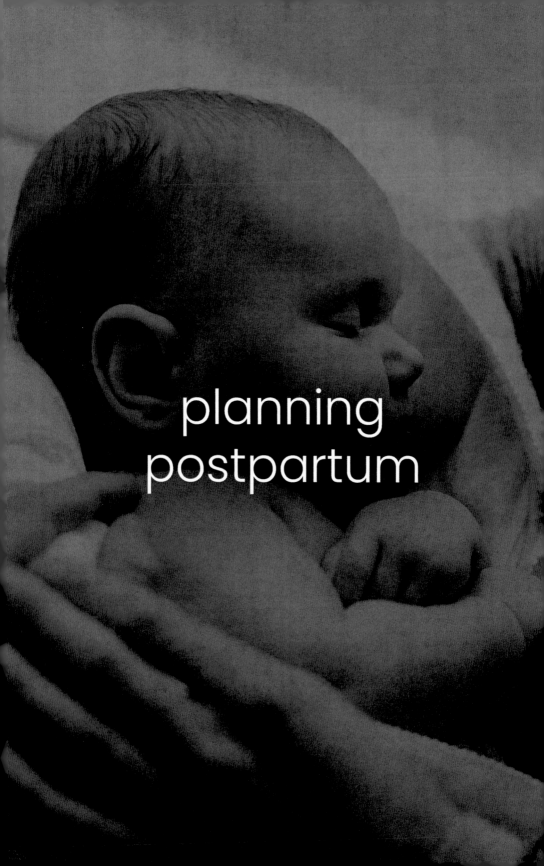

planning
postpartum

Planning Postpartum

Welcome to this space, Mama. Here we will discover how you can create your own postpartum journey with maximum support so your transition into parenthood can be as smooth as possible.

Postpartum time for new mothers can bring up some feelings of stress, anxiety, and unexpected fears. Can you plan and find all the resources you will need to have a restful, healing experience for you? Because a more intentionally planned postpartum experience will also help you build a deeper connection and intimacy with your baby, your partner, and most importantly, yourself.

Women's health expert and bestselling author Kimberly Ann Johnson in her book "The Fourth Trimester," shares her experience after giving birth:

> *"As disheartening as my symptoms were, I was even more perplexed by the lack of resources available to assist my healing. My midwives were either too busy, at a loss for how to help, or in denial about the severity of my situation to assist me in any real way."*

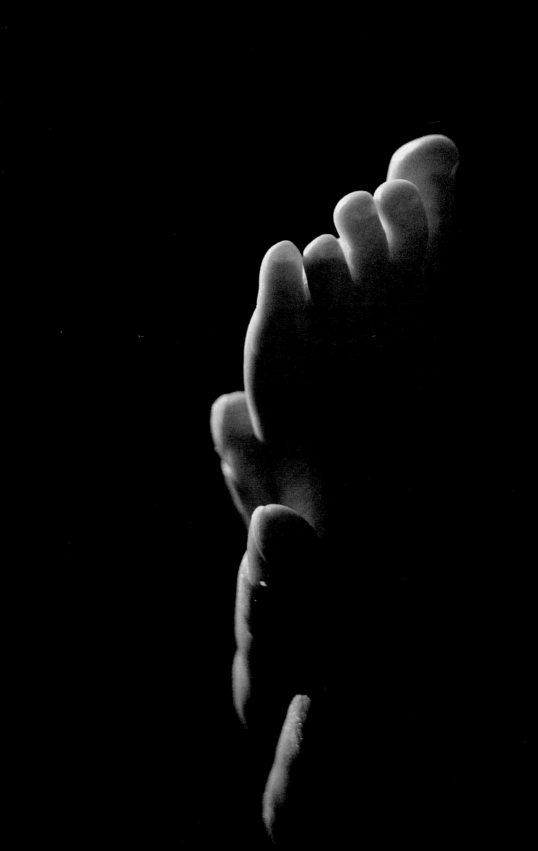

Most mothers claim that "nobody ever told them what bringing up a baby involved" and say they had to learn everything "the hard way." While it is true that the experience is individual, considering the number of courses and groups dedicated to "preparing for childbirth," I find it surprising that there are still women who reach motherhood emotionally helpless and unprepared...

Maternity, Coming face to face with our shadow, *Laura Gutman*

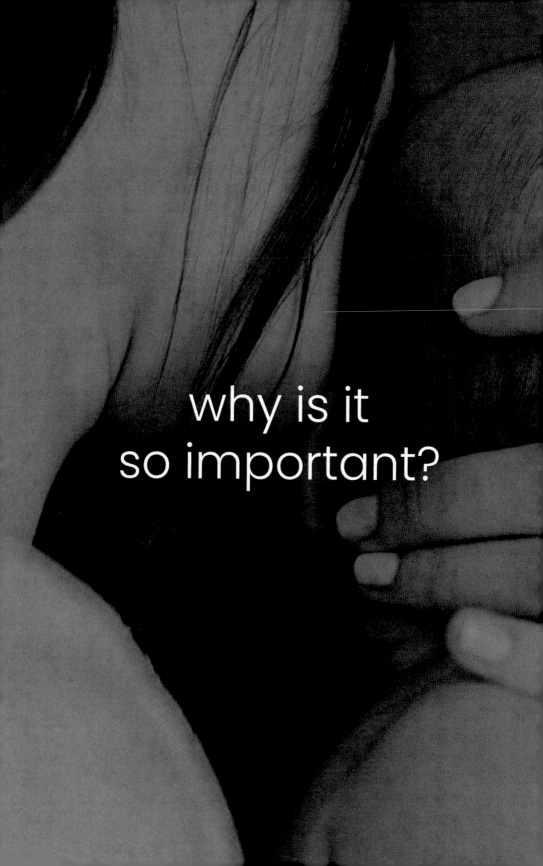

why is it
so important?

Why Is It So Important?

In reality, there is a great lack of importance placed on postpartum care in many western countries.

In many Asian countries, preparation and postpartum care is the whole community's responsibility. In the United States, however, it is seen as the sole responsibility of a future mother.

But you don't have to go through it alone. This Guide is the very first step towards creating your postpartum time to be as optimal as possible. You will learn how you can **invite your community to support you.**

The time after having a baby is one of the most vulnerable seasons of your life. How prepared you are for the time after birth will depend on your **proactive planning** and how well you **engage and educate your community.**

After reading this Guide, you can schedule a private planning session with me to further develop your support system.

Please invite your partner, a family member, or a friend you can rely on for support in practical ways to join us in the planning session.

Thoughtful and intentional planning for your support may significantly impact the trajectory of your motherhood journey.

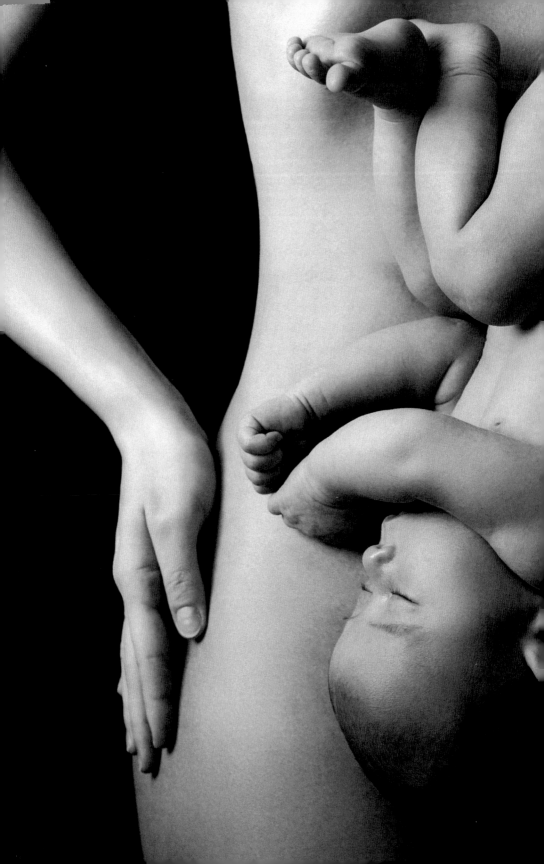

"

The idea of the fourth trimester that includes a period of forty days spent resting, nurturing ourselves, and letting others nurture us, challenges our deeply held cultural tropes of individualism and self-sufficiency, some of our feminist ideals, and our personal expectations that we are unstoppable superwomen.

"

The Fourth Trimester,
Kimberly Ann Johnson

postpartum
care for
the mother

Postpartum Care For The Mother

As mentioned earlier, the postpartum period is often called the fourth trimester, implying that the continuum of pregnancy is not over after childbirth. The three trimesters require the **fourth trimester** of postpartum care to **complete the process for both the mother and the baby.**

Therefore, postpartum care is an especially important part of the whole journey: pregnancy, birth, and care that allows you to complete the process of becoming a mother.

We are always excited to meet and talk with expecting moms and parents. They often anticipate the newest family member's arrival and make necessary plans to have the birth experience they desire.

They create a special space in their homes and accumulate all the necessary accouterments for the new baby. Their Baby Registry is full of cute baby outfits, toys, diapering gear, baby bottles, car seats, and carriers. All the necessary gear is shared with everyone as desired gifts for a new family.

> *The Traditional Baby Shower Baby showers bring family and community together before a birth; yet these social gatherings are a remnant of more meaningful rituals originally designed to help women prepare for the self-transformation that occurs during birth.*

Ancient Maps, *Pam England*

Many parents plan an elaborate **Baby Shower** where the guests bring a lot of gifts for the baby: burping rags, cute little socks, creative bibs, and other amazing things.

But one important thing is missing.

As a mother of four who now supports postpartum families in adjusting to life with a newborn, such Baby Showers often leave me heartbroken. Is there a way to create a more meaningful way and bring rituals to help initiate a new mother into motherhood?

I keep asking myself: in all of this planning, preparation, shower festivities, and shopping, what are the ceremonies that, as a community, we can gift the birthing mother with?

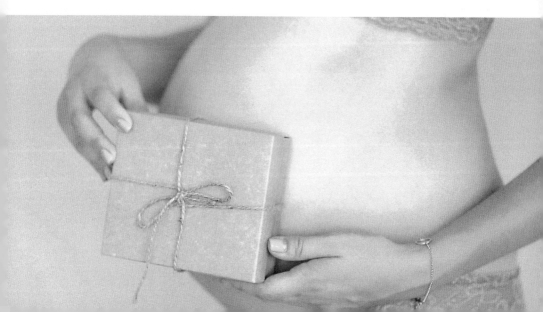

...having your body, mind, and spirit rearranged is an overhaul that requires the utmost respect and attention...I can attest that preparing the environment you will be recovering in so it nurtures this transition is the first step toward a strong beginning of your family. You will need maturity, foresight, and courage. For you'll have to go against what our culture currently says: that a fast recovery will earn you the label of Superwoman. You may be called selfish or spoiled. You may actually feel selfish or spoiled. But it starts here, with honoring the magnitude of what it is to birth a child into the world.

The Fourth Trimester, *Kimberly Ann Johnson*

As a postpartum doula, I usually see the negative implications of overlooking the most transformative and vulnerable times in women's lives. So many women throughout the Western World experience postpartum depression, anxiety, and relationship challenges that arise during the first couple of months after the baby is born.

Many new mothers during the first weeks after having a baby share that they feel unsupported, depleted, lonely, and lost after the baby is born.

Can you envision a better way for yourself? How can you find assistance, ask for help, and create a supportive community in preparing for parenthood?

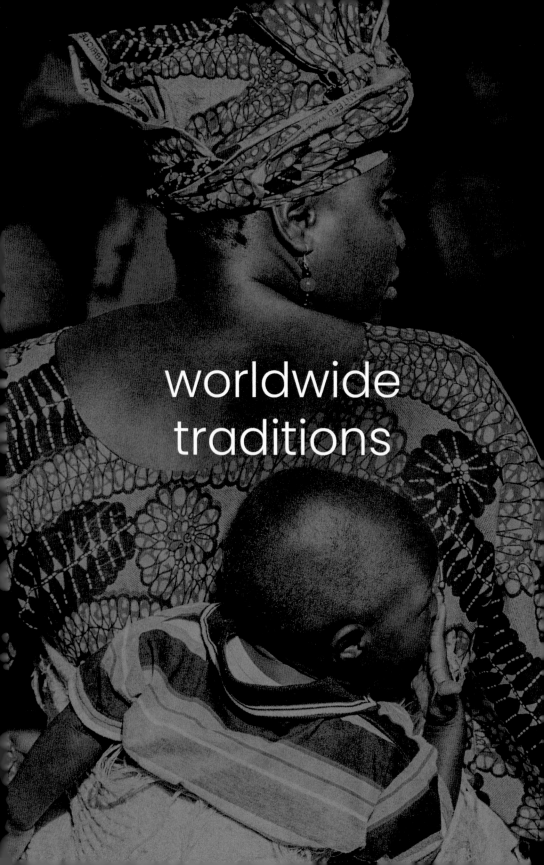

worldwide
traditions

Worldwide Traditions

> *Every pregnant woman deserves and needs to be celebrated, to feel loved and special. A birth ceremony is not optional or frivolous; it is a necessity, so mark your prenatal map of preparation with a star for "ceremony." As you prepare for your rite of passage, step out of your busy life and commit to a time and place to be honored by those close to you.*

Ancient Maps, *Pam England*

Throughout the world, in India, China, Korea, Thailand, Vietnam, Cambodia, Pakistan, Nepal, Japan, Indonesia, Jordan, Egypt, Guatemala, Mexico, Morocco, Kenya, and South Africa people have postpartum traditions that are still alive and practiced regularly.

They gather as a village around the mother, holding her through the fourth trimester, the sacred window called in India, by offering certain conditions to support healing and health.

These cultures share the same main principles for postpartum care and healing. We can call them **universal principles**.

Here are the universal principles of postpartum wellness and healing that are observed in many countries and cultures around the world:

- **Time**
- **Warmth**
- **Bodywork**
- **Rest**
- **Nourishing food**
- **Community support**

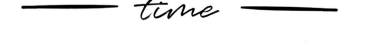

time

A time of rest that varies from three weeks to over three months. Often, it equals 40 days period).

While a new family is resting and healing postpartum, the community provides physical support such as cooking, doing laundry, shopping, cleaning, helping with older children, and running errands for the new family.

In this country, it is very different. However, usually, people in the community around expectant mothers want to help, but they do not know how. And the mothers, most of the time, do not know how or what to ask for.

This Guide is here to help you to bridge this gap. Because with the right preparation, you can start creating a supportive community that will help you to rest and heal physically, mentally, and emotionally. The first weeks in the fourth trimester must be dedicated to your **self-care, wellness, and mindfulness**. You will then be better at navigating parenting and motherhood.

Above all, postpartum care through the community offers mothering wisdom, emotional support, laughter, loving presence, and intentional consideration of the vulnerability and fragility you and your baby experience during this special time.

If there are postpartum community groups in your local area (preferably not virtual), seek them out before your baby comes. There are lactation support groups and playgroups that exist in birth centers. Look them up and connect before your baby arrives. Seek out the resources your community offers to help you thrive and promote good physical, mental, spiritual, and emotional health.

Later, in the **Guided Workbook**, you will be able to create a step-by-step process to help you **mobilize and empower your fourth-trimester community of support.**

— 66 —

Slowly it dawned on me that there was something about having others near and helpful that might be essential to successful lactation. I began to work on the idea that if breastfeeding is to succeed there must be someone around to mother the mother.

77 —

Only Mothers know, *Dana Raphael*

—— *warmth* ——

In many Asian cultures, the mother and the baby are fiercely protected from the cold, from any winds or draughts that can enter through the open windows or doors.

In Kazakhstan, where I am from, the cold is considered the enemy of health. Therefore, the new moms are given only warm, cozy clothes; they have wool scarves wrapped around their breasts and bellies. The family serves them only warm hearty soups and teas.

Also, I remember how in Kazakhstan, that during sickness, little children are rubbed with warming animal lards to allow the heat to enter the body and promote healing and the flow of energy. Special attention is given to the care of the body through relaxing or very vigorous, warming massages, oil rubs, and fire-infused cupping, including the stomach area.

In the USA, however, massage therapists are not trained in the art of belly massage, so you may be better supported by hiring a postpartum specialist, like a postpartum doula, who is trained to provide you with this type of wellness service. **Remember, having postpartum care is not a luxury but a necessity.**

massage
Bodywork

Belly binding, such as warm oil massages in India, belly massages in Mexico, or Mayan abdominal massages in Guatemala, are focused on womb care and administered to the new moms. These practices help create feelings of being grounded and safely held. During the postpartum period, we want to bring warmth to the abdomen, encourage lymph drainage, increase blood circulation, and remove toxins and excess air from the emptied womb.

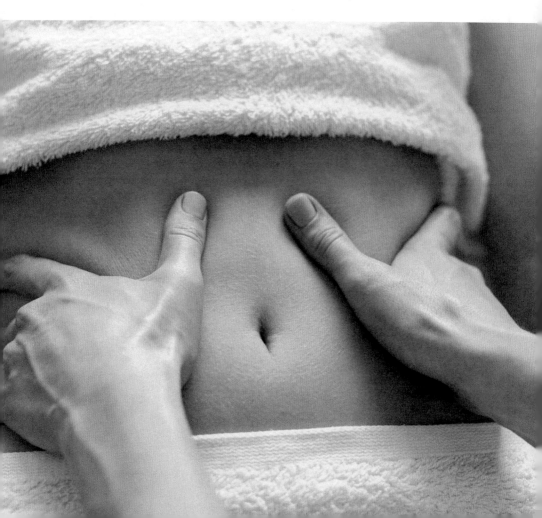

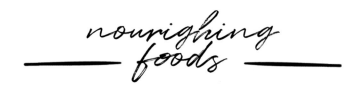

nourishing foods

Since after birth, digestion slows down, it is imperative that the meals offered to the new mother are easy to digest and nourishing. Typically soups, teas, and porridges are served until her digestion is stronger and elimination is regular and easy. As the mother's appetite and capacity to digest food grow, more dense foods are slowly introduced to provide adequate nourishment for postpartum healing and breast milk production.

In addition, if a mother chooses to breastfeed, some extra nutritional provisions will be required to support the demands of the breast milk supply.

Special postpartum massages and meals menu can be reviewed during a private one-on-one session if you decide to learn more. Together we will create a **customized meal plan** for you, which you then can share with your community to guide the design of the meal train, a service that many new families can benefit from.

Intentional massage moves the inner organs which are squished during the last months of pregnancy. Massages also encourage better blood circulation and promote energy flow for healing. I see how, like in Kazakhstan, in many indigenous countries, people grow up understanding the value of touch, but it is not as common in the United States.

If you deliver at the hospital, and your child is born at night, there may be no food available as the cafeteria is already closed. Also, many doulas have been addressing that the meals at the hospital cafeterias are unsuitable for mothers who have just delivered a baby.

In her book Ancient Maps, Pam England recommends that mothers bring herbal teas, packets of miso, nutritious salty broth, or frozen homemade soup that can be warmed up. She continues: "For the first few weeks after birth, the new mother should eat warm, easy-to-digest comfort foods such as mushy cooked whole-grain cereals, casseroles, soups, and rice and tapioca puddings."

> *Making sure you are well fed is one of the priorities of this postpartum period, and a great way to build and lean on community at this time...While there are variations in ingredients and spices from culture to culture, what the postpartum foods have in common across cultures is that they are warming, easy to digest, mineral rich, and collagen dense.*

Fourth Trimester, *Kimberly Ann Johnson*

Nourishment is also offered for the mind of the mother.

In Kazakhstan, easy "digestive" words, more silence, and whispering are heard in a new mother's home. The mother is encouraged to relax and enjoy this time with the newborn with the support of family and friends caring for them. They are discouraged from experiencing worry or stress about anything. The family and friends protect a new mom from negativity, bad news, or anything else disturbing her peace.

Think of this protective emotional field when you choose your village. Who can help you create and support it? Could it be your mother or mother-in-law? Can they offer you this nourishment? Or your partner? Think of those people that you can add to your **Guided Workbook**.

In addition to building your village with friends and family, you may consider hiring a trained **postpartum doula**, who supports you with no agenda or judgment and will give you important unbiased care and nurturing during this time.

> *A woman during postpartum should not be left on her own for long. She needs the help, companionship, and availability of another person who will not interfere or abuse her authority or be meddlesome but who is simply present. They must take responsibility for all tasks which can be delegated, caring for older children, cleaning, preparing meals, shopping, and washing the clothes of the mother with a baby in her arms, and organizing the household while attending to the unspoken needs.*

Maternity, Coming Face To Face With Your Shadow,
Laura Gutman

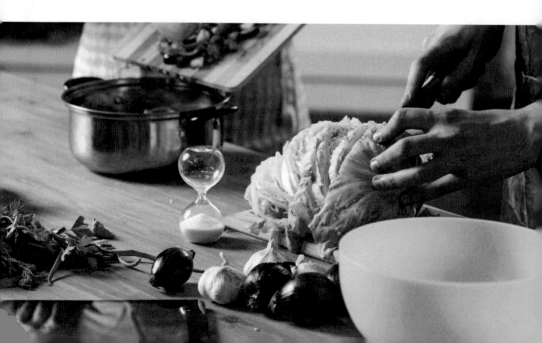

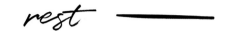

rest

Rest is another particularly vital component of postpartum care. It absolutely does not mean that you must sleep all the time.

For many women in America, rest may mean being in passive, sleeping mode. Rather, rest in postpartum means an unhurried way of being. It can especially refer to a certain mindset that is free of thoughts and not preoccupied with various to-do lists.

Ideally, this is the time **when you are not in a rush and savoring each moment of discovering who you are becoming**. You focus on spending time with the baby, feeding yourself and the baby, and enjoying the nourishment you both receive.

Creating supportive practices to encourage resting and tending to your own health can include taking relaxing baths, doing healing steaming rituals, journaling, and meditating. Your healing body can benefit from rejuvenating movements such as postpartum yoga, Feldenkrais, and gentle pilates.

If you have a **postpartum doula**, she can hold and feed the baby while you nap. A visiting friend may allow you to rest, shower, and do your laundry. Think of some names you can add to the **Guided Workbook**.

Can your partner take the baby for a walk outside and let you relax for an hour or two? This all requires planning and strong and clear communication on your part. You can also flesh all this out during our group planning sessions.

Remember, people are usually happy to help and be useful to you when they are visiting. However, they will not guess or read your mind and most likely will feel lost and not know what may be helpful to you. You can share with them what is needed and what is supportive for you during this time. **You are helping them when you let them know how to help you. And imagine how you can receive their help.**

— **"**

Patience and perspective allow you and your partner to fully integrate the social, emotional, and physical changes, as well as your new identity as parents.

"

Ancient Maps, *Pam England*, p.610

community support

In some Asian cultures, and even in some communities in the US, there are exclusive luxury postpartum hotels where new mothers can check in and have all their needs met by a dedicated staff member, utilizing all the postpartum healing traditions.

While in this country, most mothers do not have this option available, can you imagine what a postpartum healing hotel would ideally look and feel like for you? What are the five most essential elements of this option that are specifically important to you? Can you re-create this in your home? Hopefully, you can now recognize that the most important nursery to set up before your baby's birth is a postpartum **nursery for yourself**.

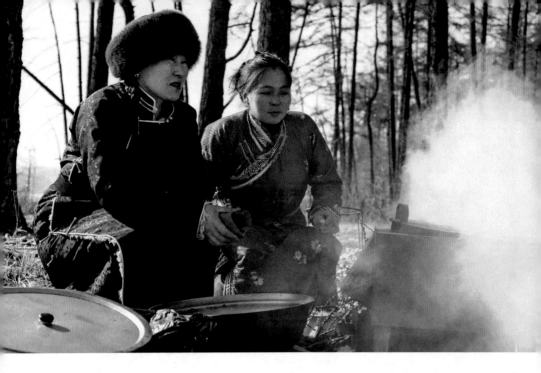

For example, think of some people among your friends and family who can help you organize the nursery that considers your optimal postpartum healing.

With community support comes another necessity - **creating appropriate boundaries**. Will you have certain hours that visitors can come? Is there a list of things you will ask them to help you with while they are visiting?

Consider setting clear boundaries with visitors who can hold a newborn and when? Maybe not having anyone over before the baby is at least a week old. Is it okay if they put their fingers in the baby's mouth?

What will the people visiting you need to be aware of to foster and promote a special atmosphere of nurturing and caring for your well-being?

You can start exploring these ideas now and discuss them with your partner. Remember to discuss these with your postpartum doula if you hire one.

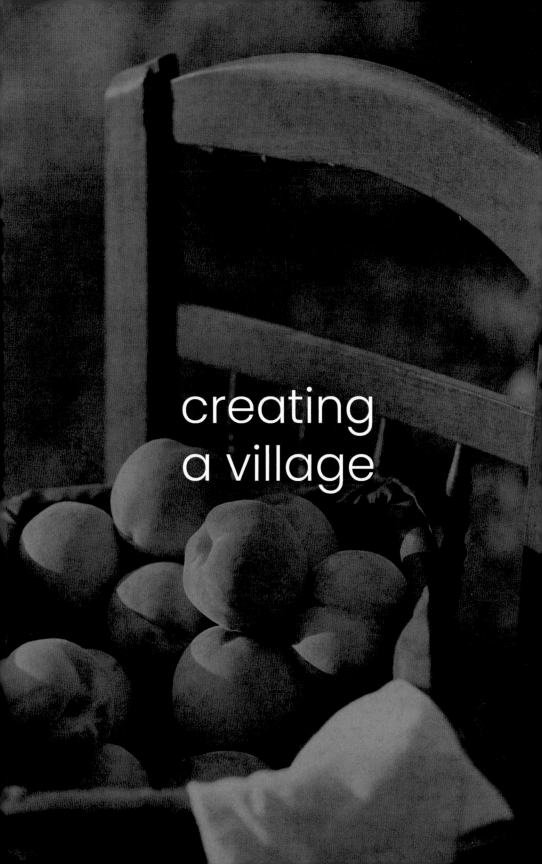

creating
a village

Creating A Village

We are social creatures; we are not supposed to be left alone after we give birth to our babies. I see this as feelings of isolation that new mothers experience during the postpartum window.

In the Western world, there is a great resurgence and realization of the need to **re-create villages around new mothers** to provide the support they need. The new mothers and the family as a whole need support as they all go through the transition together.

Closeness and the right emotional support of another human being, without any judgment or expectations of the lactating woman, diminishes the levels of stress and anxiety, which in turn support healthy levels of the hormones responsible for milk supply.

Dana Raphael, an anthropologist, coined the term, **Doula**. She studied breastfeeding in other cultures and noticed that to ensure successful breastfeeding, it is important to have a supportive person around the new mother during the first weeks postpartum. Birth and Postpartum **Doulas** are trained people who support women during and after birth.

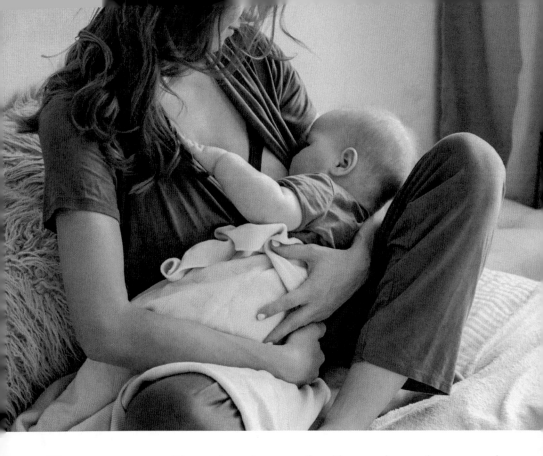

The postpartum village that the new family needs can be created through intentional planning. Think through and choose carefully who will be allowed or invited to be there for you, to hold and care for your family through the transition. This is just the beginning of a new life for you as a mother. You and your community can make it more enjoyable and give a healthy start through postpartum planning.

As a postpartum educator, I am here to guide you and your community to know how we can help your family keep the household running smoothly while you recover and bond with you newborn baby.

If you have an expecting mother as your friend or a neighbor, consider including a thoughtful gift for the mother during the baby shower. Please connect with me to learn more.

Your family and friends can give you a monetary gift to help hire necessary support, including a postpartum doula. I partner with a service-based Gift Registry called Be Her Village, which you can check out.

Can the whole family pitch in and give the mother the most needed time and rest she will need after the birth is over?

As a mother, what do you do regularly to ensure you feel at ease while you heal and stay off your feet for 4-6 weeks following a vaginal birth and longer with a cesarean birth (8 weeks)?

In the **Journal**, list any household caring needs: dishes, laundry, babysitting, meal preparation, groceries, and all the tasks you typically take care of that will need to be delegated. During our Planning Session, you will add the names of those who can assist with those tasks.

journal

Let's Make It Practical

In this Journal, you will have a "brain dump" session! Think of the things you would like to be taken care of while you are snuggling with your baby.

These instructions will help your visitors feel empowered and informed about how to do things for you independently and not bother you if you are taking a much-needed nap or shower.

What are your top priorities to feel at ease at home? This may include having a clean kitchen, swept floors, having laundry put away, having the groceries delivered, and having the meals planned.

_____

_____

_____

_____

_____

_____

_____

Kitchen: where the groceries go (label shelves and cupboards).

_____

_____

_____

Laundry: label drawers and shelves for where to sort your laundry, place labels for what detergent and which setting on the washer and dryer should be used.

_____

_____

_____

_____

_____

Now, list those special people with the gifts to help you with all these chores.

_____

_____

_____

_____

_____

How would you like to communicate this to them? If you hire a postpartum doula, she may reach out to them on your behalf and help organize it. You may also ask your best friend to do it. Think of it as something the maid of honor would be helping with at the wedding. We can discuss more at our session.

_____

_____

_____

_____

_____

What are the things that your partner or parents can help you with? Take the older siblings out? Take the baby once a day for a 30-minute walk?

_____

_____

_____

_____

_____

What are some "me-time" activities you want to prioritize within the first 6 - 8 weeks postpartum? Take a relaxing shower, drink herbal teas, and get a massage every week or daily.

_____

_____

_____

_____

_____

_____

_____

_____

_____

_____

_____

_____

Mama-friendly movement: What would you like to start with? Gentle yoga? Or a daily walk outside?

_____

_____

_____

_____

_____

_____

_____

_____

_____

_____

_____

_____

Mindfulness: 10 minutes of meditation and breathwork daily can help you reduce stress, control your emotions, and clear your head. Also, limiting social media would be considered a wellness activity. Think and promise yourself to cultivate these to promote your healing.

_____

_____

_____

_____

_____

_____

_____

_____

_____

_____

_____

_____

_____

Community: Who are the people with whom you can have life-giving conversations that leave you feeling rejuvenated? No drama-people, please. They are great to come, make you warm tea, and listen without judgment. This is nourishment for your soul.

_____

_____

_____

_____

_____

_____

_____

_____

_____

_____

_____

_____

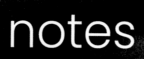

notes

Notes

guided
workbook

With this **Guidebook**, you are creating a resource for your postpartum doula or best friend. You can share this guidebook and together with your partner, husband, or a close friend create a spreadsheet, putting in their names and the ways your community can support you.

putting it
all together

Putting It All Together

Our Community/Our Village

Think and choose people who you would feel comfortable asking to clean your toilet and who you would feel comfortable being vulnerable with, who you feel completely safe with and would be comfortable being totally honest with. It's ideal if there is at least one of each of your support people who is local and will be able to lend a physical hand, however if that is not possible, list your virtual support and we will brainstorm additional resources who may fill in the gaps like a postpartum doula, massage therapist, personal chef, mother's helper, etc. The professional people might also be additional people in your outer layers of support.

1. Name: _____
Phone number: _____
Email address:
Availability: _____
What can i ask of this person?
_____
_____

2. Name: _____
Phone number: _____
Email address:
Availability: _____
What can i ask of this person?
_____
_____

3. Name: _____
Phone number: _____
Email address:
Availability: _____
What can i ask of this person?
_____
_____

4. Name: _____
Phone number: _____
Email address:
Availability: _____
What can i ask of this person?
_____
_____

Our outer layers of support:

Who would be happy to support you but who you might not want in your innermost circle of support? Here are some possible tasks your outer layer of support can help with either right away or further along in your postpartum healing:

Meal train (Postpartum friendly, Ayurvedic meals):

_____

_____

Bulk food prep (Girlfriends Party to make and freeze meals for a mama?)

_____

_____

Picking up groceries: (list of postpartum-friendly foods)

_____

_____

Running an errand:

_____

_____

Walking your dog:

_____

_____

Playdates with your older children:

_____

_____

Other ways your community can help out and who would you want
to help in this way?

_____

_____

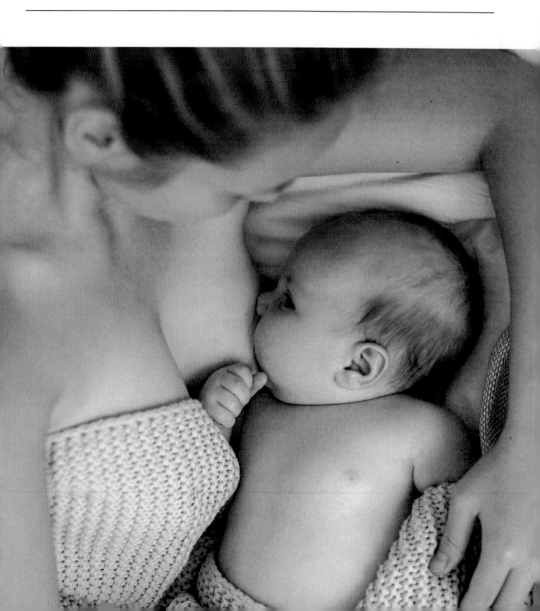

Professional Support

Sometimes a little extra support is needed and incredibly helpful.

Postpartum Doula:

*Would you want to be specific about what you'd want more of?
Household help and cooking? Wellness and massages? Emotional
support? While postpartum doulas are trained in all of these areas, they
still may have their own strengths and preferences. Most importantly,
when you interview your future doula, listen to yourself: do you feel
safe and relaxed with her? Does she help you release stress and anxiety?
Postpartum is a very vulnerable space for you to be. And you want
someone you are completely safe with to be there.*

_____

_____

_____

_____

_____

Overnight Doula/Newborn Care specialist

_____

_____

_____

_____

_____

Babysitters/Nanny's for older children

Finding a right fit and a reliable person can take time. Also, your older children will need some time to get used to that person, who will understand the magnitude of the transition the whole family will be going through with a newborn coming home with you. So when you interview a babysitter or nanny ask a few questions that will allow you and the other person who you are interviewing to consider the specifics of the postpartum time.

_____

_____

_____

_____

_____

Lactation Consultant:

_____

_____

_____

_____

_____

Postpartum Support Group:

_____

_____

_____

_____

_____

Mental Health Support:

_____

_____

_____

_____

_____

Mommy and Me playgroups:

_____

_____

_____

_____

_____

Other Professional Support:

_____

_____

_____

_____

_____

House Cleaners:

_____

_____

_____

_____

_____

Massage Therapists:

_____

_____

_____

_____

_____

Chiropractors:

_____

_____

_____

_____

_____

Craniosacral Therapists (for you and the newborn)

_____

_____

_____

_____

_____

Pelvic Floor Practitioners:

_____

_____

_____

_____

_____

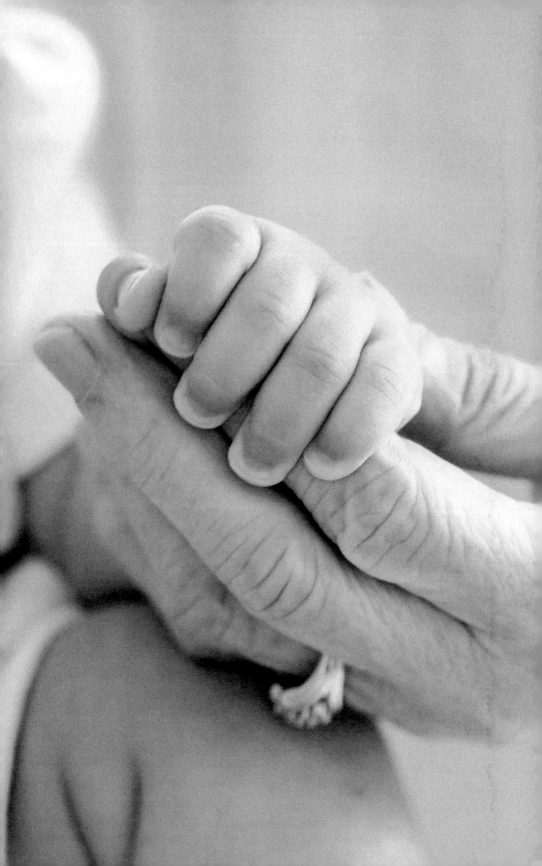

planning
session

After Birth Well-being Planning Session

If you would like to go further in planning and organizing your postpartum care and healing time, to create for yourself an opportunity, a space, and allow the time to heal, to connect with your baby, as well as transition to your new role and identity with less stress and anxiety, please schedule a postpartum planning session.

You will go through a range of emotions that you have never experienced, sometimes all in one day. You will experience periods of doubt. You will need companionship that you can rely on, assuring you that everything is okay, that you will reemerge... I have never heard a woman lament having too much postpartum support. I have only heard women regret that no one told them they should have invested more resources in postpartum care.

Fourth Trimester, *Kimberly Ann Johnson*

During our **Planning Session,** you will:

- clarify what needs you will have after you have a newborn
- what items you can add to your Baby Registry to benefit you too
- how to set up a baby nursery that will also satisfy your needs
- how hormonal changes will affect your wellbeing
- meal planning that takes into consideration the specificity of the postpartum digestion
- how you can mobilize your community to support you effectively

...and many other elements will help you better prepare for the most transformative and vulnerable season of your life!

Schedule a private Planning Session with Zaure
www.pamperingdoula.com

Schedule a private Planning Session with Ashlee
www.lifenectar.com

Made in the USA
Monee, IL
03 March 2023

28463797R00045